An Introduction to the Joint Commission

Its Survey and Accreditation Processes, Standards, and Services

Joint Commission on Accreditation of Hospitals

An Introduction to the Joint Commission

Its Survey and Accreditation Processes, Standards, and Services

Joint Commission on Accreditation of Hospitals

Prepared by the Department of Publications
Barbara Brandt, Project Editor
Mary Ann Simmonds, Designer

875 North Michigan Avenue, Chicago, Illinois 60611
First edition published 1985. Second edition 1987.

ISBN: 0-86688-120-4
Library of Congress Catalog Card Number: 86-83310

Foreword

The Joint Commission on Accreditation of Hospitals is a private, not-for-profit organization dedicated to improving the quality of care in organized health care settings through voluntary accreditation. Since it was founded in 1951, the Joint Commission has become the principal standards setter for health care organizations – not only for hospitals, but also for long term care organizations, hospice programs, ambulatory health care organizations, psychiatric organizations, and other programs.

The Joint Commission's role has been dynamic, involving the continual adaptation of its standards and accreditation and survey processes to the evolving health care field and the society of which it is a part. New concepts in care (such as hospice programs and emergicenters), new organizational approaches to health care (such as multi-institutional systems), the increasing numbers of elderly people, the concern for managing costs while maintaining quality, the advances made in science and medical technology – these and many other issues are changing the nature, delivery, and settings of health care.

Constant throughout these changes, however, has been the Joint Commission's commitment to improving the quality of health care. In 1986 the Joint Commission adopted an "agenda for change" to launch a new era for quality assurance in health care; some of the elements of this multifaceted initiative are described in this book. One particularly important effort is the expansion and enhancement of the Joint Commission's role as educator and consultant. Through improved education programs, publications, consultation, and other activities, the Joint Commission assures the availability of resource support for those who desire to provide high-quality health services.

This book presents an overview of the Joint Commission, its accreditation process, and its services. Chapter 1 examines the concept of voluntary accreditation – its history, development through the years, and significance in today's health care world. Chapter 2 discusses the Joint Commission's survey and accreditation processes – the way surveys are conducted, the factors that affect accreditation decisions, and recent developments in the accreditation process. Chapter 3 is about Joint Commission standards – how they are developed and what kinds of changes in health care influence their development. Finally, Chapter 4 describes the resources and services that the Joint Commission makes available to health care organizations.

We at the Joint Commission hope that this guide will help to foster an increased awareness and appreciation of the role that voluntary accreditation plays in maintaining and improving the quality of health care provided in this country. The request of an organization for a Joint Commission survey represents a voluntary commitment to evaluation and self-improvement. We invite all health care organizations to avail themselves of the many services that the Joint Commission offers.

Dennis S. O'Leary, MD
President

CONTENTS

Chapter 1

VOLUNTARY ACCREDITATION

Its Significance and Evolution in A Changing Health Care Environment

Through its voluntary accreditation process, the Joint Commission on Accreditation of Hospitals strives to meet the needs of a changing health care environment by developing national standards that reflect consensus on the state of the art, by conducting on-site surveys of organizations that voluntarily seek accreditation, and by awarding accreditation to organizations that substantially meet the standards. The mission of the Joint Commission is both to assist health care organizations in complying with its standards and to assess the level of compliance they have achieved. To ensure that voluntary accreditation remains a viable force for promoting the quality of care in health care organizations, the Joint Commission conducts its educational and accreditation activities with attention to changing practices in health care and current trends in health care delivery.

Current Trends in Health Care

During the past several years, many significant changes have occurred in the nature, delivery, and settings of health care. The growing elderly segment of the population, the development of new organizational approaches to the delivery of services (such as multi-institutional systems), the increasingly severe cost constraints that make the effort to maintain quality all the more imperative – these are but a few of the issues affecting health care today. The Joint Commission takes these and other issues into account when it revises its standards and its survey and accreditation processes.

Today's health care system is characterized by economic competition, resource limitations, and new delivery systems – of which a significant number are unmonitored. It is more important now than ever before to promote high-quality care, and the Joint Commission continues to do so by developing standards intended to assure that patients receive the care and services they need, including continuity of care within and across health care settings. In response to the increasing variety of health care organizations, the Joint Commission has tailored its survey process to meet the specific needs of diverse organizations. For example, for hospitals that have 100,000 or more outpatient visits per year, an ambulatory health care surveyor is added to the survey team. And, in recognition of the growing multi-institutional segment of the health care field, the Joint Commission participated in a study of multihospital systems, which resulted in revised standards and the option of a modified survey process for such systems and their constituent organizations. The Joint Commission is now studying multi-institutional systems in other health care settings, such as long term care.

By addressing health care trends, the Joint Commission continues to help maintain and improve the quality of care provided by our nation's health care organizations. A survey process that evolves in response to the current health care environment enhances the viability and significance of voluntary accreditation.

The Significance of Voluntary Accreditation

Joint Commission accreditation is voluntary. The decision to be surveyed is made by the individuals who are responsible for operating an organization. This voluntary aspect is of crucial importance because it indicates that an organization has voluntarily sought to be measured against national, professionally based standards for health care and services, has been found to be in substantial compliance with the standards, and is making an effort to provide even better care and services.

The accreditation process allows health care organizations to

- achieve consensus, through the standards development process, on elements essential to high-quality care;
- identify deficiencies in performance;
- benefit from external evaluation, education, and consultation;
- document the organization's accountability for effective and efficient operation; and
- take advantage of interinstitutional comparisons and exchanges.

The Joint Commission's role is one not only of evaluator but also of educator and consultant. Its accreditation and survey processes are dedicated to identifying an organization's strengths and weaknesses and to providing assistance in correcting the identified weaknesses. For example, at the end of a survey, Joint Commission surveyors meet with representatives of an organization to discuss preliminary findings and to make suggestions for improvement. The survey report that accompanies each accreditation decision details an organization's deficiencies and includes recommendations for correcting them and for raising the level of staff performance. If an organization is accredited with one or more contingencies, the Joint Commission offers additional guidance until the organization is able to demonstrate improvement in the area or areas of concern.

The Joint Commission publishes numerous educational materials, conducts a variety of seminars throughout the country, and provides consultation related to accreditation and technical assistance regarding other quality of care concerns of health care professionals who request such support. In addition, Joint Commission standards provide guidelines for organizations to use in developing and maintaining continuing education and self-evaluation programs.

The Joint Commission's national reputation for promoting high-quality health care has led some regulatory agencies to consider its accreditation decisions as a factor in granting certification and/or licensure. Similarly, some insurance carriers are influenced by Joint Commission accreditation decisions in honoring reimbursement claims. In addition, the federal government has given recognition to Joint Commission hospital accreditation in its Medicare legislation. However, it should be emphasized that the Joint Commission supports the private initiative in health care, promotes the voluntary aspect of accreditation, and strives to protect the confidentiality of information obtained through the accreditation survey process.

To understand the significance of voluntary accreditation and the directions it is likely to take in the future, it is helpful to understand how voluntary accreditation began and how it has changed through the years.

How Voluntary Accreditation Began

The Joint Commission's voluntary hospital accreditation program originated in 1913 with the American College of Surgeons (ACS). The College members believed that some system of standardization of hospitals and hospital work should be developed, and in 1915 they allocated $500 to establish standards for promoting high-quality patient care in hospitals. By 1917, with the financial assistance of the Carnegie Foundation, the ACS had compiled a one-page list of requirements, called the *Minimum Standard for Hospitals.*

In 1918 the ACS instituted a program to conduct on-site inspections of hospitals having more than 100 beds. In the first year the program was offered, almost 700 hospitals were inspected, but only 89 met the requirements of the *Minimum Standard.* These statistics, which the ACS released without naming the hospitals that had been inspected, made the American medical community keenly aware of the need for the ACS standards. With the support of the medical community, ACS accreditation became a widely accepted means of maintaining and improving the quality of care. By 1951 voluntary accreditation had proved its value to the health care field; more than 3,000 hospitals had been voluntarily surveyed and had met the *Minimum Standard.*

The Joint Commission on Accreditation of Hospitals

The success of the hospital standardization program made it impossible for the ACS to continue to support it alone, and other national professional organizations were invited to participate. Thus, in 1951, the American College of Physicians, the American Medical Association, the Canadian Medical Association, and the American Hospital Association joined with the ACS to form the Joint Commission on Accreditation of Hospitals. The Canadian Medical Association withdrew to form its own national accrediting organization in 1959, and the American Dental Association joined the Joint Commission in 1980. Through the years, the member organizations have helped shape Joint Commission policy through the representatives they appoint to the Board of Commissioners, the Joint Commission's governing body.

Today, the Joint Commission is governed by 22 commissioners, 21 of whom are appointed by the five member organizations. In 1981 the Board of Commissioners appointed its first public member to provide a perspective on consumer concerns.

The Board meets three times a year to examine current issues relating to the standards and survey process for the Joint Commission's five accreditation programs: the Accreditation Program for Ambulatory Health Care, the Accreditation Program for Hospice Care, the Hospital Accreditation Program, the Accreditation Program for Long Term Care, and the Accreditation Program for Psychiatric Facilities.

The Accreditation Programs

History and Development

The Joint Commission's first voluntary accreditation program began surveying hospitals in 1952. By 1965 the Hospital Accreditation Program had gained national scope and acceptance, and the Board of Commissioners began to consider the need for voluntary accreditation programs for health care organizations other than hospitals. Accordingly, over the following decade, the Joint Commission developed survey and accreditation services for long term care organizations; for ambulatory health care organizations; and for psychiatric services, alcoholism and drug abuse programs, community mental health service programs, and programs for the mentally retarded/developmentally disabled.

The Accreditation Program for Hospice Care was established in 1983 after an extensive 2½-year study of hospice organizations in the United States. With funding from the WK Kellogg Foundation of Battle Creek, Michigan, the Joint Commission initiated the study in recognition of the growing importance of hospice care. During the project, standards and a self-assessment and survey process for hospice programs were developed, and in January 1984, the nation's first accreditation program for hospice care began conducting surveys.

The Joint Commission began a similar project in 1986 in response to the rapidly growing home care services industry. Home care has become a viable, cost-effective alternative to hospitalization or other institutionalization, particularly for the elderly. Cost-containment pressures in inpatient care encourage the prompt discharge of patients whose needs for continuing care may be met in other settings, such as the home; and technological advances have made it possible to provide a greater variety of treatments in patients' homes. The increased attention to home care has prompted concerns about the quality of home care services, which, together with the concerns raised by payers, community-based home care providers, and other health care professionals, have indicated a need for national standards. The comprehensive standards and survey process developed through the Joint Commission's project will apply to all types of organizations providing home care services, including hospital-based agencies, proprietary agencies, and community non-profit agencies. The accreditation process for home care services will become available in January 1988.

Program Information

In order to accommodate a wide range of health care organizations, the Joint Commission offers the following accreditation programs:

- The Accreditation Program for Ambulatory Health Care;
- The Accreditation Program for Hospice Care;
- The Accreditation Program for Long Term Care;
- The Accreditation Program for Psychiatric Facilities; and
- The Hospital Accreditation Program.

Each of these accreditation programs was established to encourage the provision of high-quality patient care through a peer-based consultative and educational survey process. For all of the organizations that voluntarily seek accreditation through these programs, accreditation provides a motivational force for continued self-improvement and represents a commitment to quality care.

Accreditation Program for Ambulatory Health Care. The following types of ambulatory health care organizations and programs are eligible for accreditation by the Joint Commission:

- Ambulatory surgery centers;
- Armed services clinics;
- College and university health programs;
- Community health centers;
- Emergency care centers;
- Family practice centers;
- Health maintenance organizations;
- Multispecialty group practices;
- Primary care centers;
- Single-specialty group practices; and
- Urgent care centers.

The Joint Commission uses the *Ambulatory Health Care Standards Manual* to survey ambulatory health care organizations.

Accreditation Program for Hospice Care. The Accreditation Program for Hospice Care was established to encourage the provision of high-quality care for terminally ill patients and their families. The Joint Commission surveys and accredits all types of hospice care providers, including

- independent programs;
- hospital-based programs;
- programs that are a service of a home health agency;
- programs that are a service of a long term care organization; and
- programs that are a service of a psychiatric organization.

To be eligible for survey, a hospice program must offer interdisciplinary team services at home and in inpatient settings. Interdisciplinary team services include physician, nursing, psychological/social work, spiritual, and bereavement services. Hospice programs are surveyed with the *Hospice Standards Manual.*

Accreditation Program for Long Term Care. The Accreditation Program for Long Term Care surveys both hospital-based and freestanding long term care organizations. More than 1,300 long term care organizations are currently accredited under the *Long Term Care Standards Manual.*

Accreditation Program for Psychiatric Facilities. The Joint Commission established the Accreditation Program for Psychiatric Facilities to encourage the provision of high-quality care for patients and residents of psychiatric and/or substance abuse organizations and programs. These programs and services include

- alcoholism and substance abuse programs;
- community mental health service programs;
- forensic psychiatric services;
- programs for the mentally retarded/developmentally disabled; and
- psychiatric services.

The Joint Commission currently accredits more than 1,200 facilities, programs, and services under the *Consolidated Standards Manual.*

Hospital Accreditation Program. The Hospital Accreditation Program accredits all types of general hospitals under the nationally recognized standards in the *Accreditation Manual for Hospitals.* Approximately 5,000 of the nation's 5,800 general hospitals are accredited. Hospital-based psychiatric and substance abuse services and freestanding psychiatric and substance abuse hospitals are also surveyed and accredited through the Hospital Accreditation Program.

Each accreditation program is advised by a Professional and Technical Advisory Committee (PTAC) composed of experts in the field. Most PTAC members represent health care professional organizations active in their respective fields. The knowledge and experience of PTAC members help to ensure that the accreditation programs address current health care trends. Accreditation program and standards development staff work closely with the PTACs in establishing and refining standards and in strengthening the survey process.

In the past few years, the combined efforts of Joint Commission staff, Board members, and PTAC representatives have resulted in several important changes in Joint Commission standards and in the survey and accreditation processes, which affect all accreditation programs.

Developments in Standards and in the Accreditation Process

In 1981 the Joint Commission began a major project to revise and update its standards. The purpose of this ongoing project is both to streamline the standards and to make them flexible enough to be applicable to a variety of health care organizational structures. Standards that are more general and less prescriptive allow each organization the opportunity to achieve compliance in ways that best suit its unique needs.

After the standards revision project was underway, the Joint Commission undertook changes in its accreditation and survey processes. In 1982 the Joint Commission began to award accreditation for three years and to award accreditation with contingencies. Three-year accreditation decisions reduce the costly and time-consuming preparations for more frequent surveys, and the use of contingencies allows the Joint Commission to increase its attention (and that of the surveyed organizations) to problem areas and to monitor the organization's progress in correcting the deficiencies.

More recently, the Joint Commission designed the tailored and modified surveys previously discussed in this chapter to accommodate organizations that provide more than one kind of health care service and organizations that are part of multi-institutional systems. In 1986 the Joint Commission adopted an "agenda for change" to seek a more refined approach to the evaluation of the quality of care. While the accreditation process traditionally has focused on the structure and process of health care delivery, the agenda for change calls for the development of measurements of clinical and organizational performance. In addition, standards are being developed to address the issue of undercare and the importance of risk management activities, especially with regard to patient safety and quality assurance.

Summary

The Joint Commission's expansion and incorporation of new ideas have been necessary to keep pace with the dramatic changes in the nature, delivery, and settings of health care in the last three decades. The evolution of the Joint Commission reflects its commitment to ensuring that the voluntary accreditation process remains a viable and positive force for maintaining and improving quality in health care organizations. Through the years, the standards and the survey and accreditation processes have been strengthened and revised to reflect the state of the art in health care and related services. Standards are being restructured to focus more effectively on those elements essential to high-quality care, and the survey and accreditation processes are continuously reviewed so that they reflect the current health care environment. ■

Chapter 2

The Survey and Accreditation Processes

Because the Joint Commission is dedicated to promoting quality in many areas of health care and related human services, the evaluation processes used by its accreditation programs must be tailored to each organization's programs and services. Thus the Joint Commission's survey and accreditation processes focus on the specific needs of various types of health care organizations while still working to promote consistency among the standards and accreditation programs.

The primary purpose of a survey is to assess the extent of an organization's compliance with the Joint Commission standards that apply to the services it provides. There are five standards manuals: the *Accreditation Manual for Hospitals*, the *Ambulatory Health Care Standards Manual*, the *Consolidated Standards Manual*, the *Hospice Standards Manual*, and the *Long Term Care Standards Manual*.

Each standards manual contains a "General Administrative Policies and Procedures" section, which lists the eligibility criteria for determining which organizations may apply for a Joint Commission survey. This section also describes the process through which the Joint Commission surveys and accredits an organization.

Surveyors and Survey Teams

All Joint Commission surveyors are thoroughly trained to conduct the different types of surveys offered by the accreditation program to which they are assigned. They represent a wide variety of professional experience and are selected for an accreditation program on the basis of their training, education, and prior activities. Because survey team composition and survey requirements differ for each accreditation program, surveyor selection criteria vary from program to program.

The composition of a survey team is based on the size and type of the organization it will survey and on the services the organization provides. The Joint Commission alters the composition of teams to meet the needs of a specific organization. When a particular kind of service is provided in sufficient volume, the survey team includes surveyors who have special expertise in that service. General information about surveyors and survey teams for each accreditation program is provided below.

Accreditation Program for Ambulatory Health Care

Survey teams generally consist of at least one physician and one administrator. All surveyors are currently in active practice.

Accreditation Program for Hospice Care

The surveyors have administrative, educational, and/or clinical health care experience, often in hospice programs in a variety of settings. Hospice surveys are usually conducted by one surveyor.

Hospital Accreditation Program

For many general acute-care hospitals, the survey team consists of a physician, an administrator, a registered nurse, and a medical technologist. For a freestanding psychiatric hospital or for an organization in which more than 50% of the beds are for psychiatric or substance abuse patients, the physician surveyor is a psychiatrist. Similarly, for a freestanding rehabilitation hospital, the physician surveyor is a rehabilitation physician; for a hospital that contains a comprehensive rehabilitation program or unit, a rehabilitation physician is added to the usual survey team at the hospital's request. The Joint Commission is exploring the possibility of developing specialized teams to survey other types of hospitals with special needs.

Accreditation Program for Long Term Care

Surveys may be conducted by one or more of the following health care practitioners: nursing home administrator, registered nurse, social worker, or another professional who has appropriate training and experience. Long term care surveys are usually conducted by one surveyor.

Accreditation Program for Psychiatric Facilities

Organizations may be surveyed by one or more of the following health care professionals: psychiatrist, administrator, psychologist, registered nurse, or psychiatric social worker. For a residential alcoholism treatment center, for example, the survey might be conducted by a psychiatrist and/or another clinical practitioner with experience in the treatment of substance abuse.

A thorough education program is conducted to prepare new surveyors for their responsibilities as evaluators and consultants. Surveyor training emphasizes practical, participative learning activities, such as case studies, role playing, site visits, and preceptorships, to develop the surveyor's awareness of successful approaches to compliance with accreditation standards. The Joint Commission also provides a continuing education program that is designed to keep surveyors abreast of developments in medical technology, health care organizational structures, Joint Commission standards, and numerous other subjects that may affect the way the survey process is conducted.

Because effective surveyor performance is essential to a meaningful survey process, the Joint Commission continually evaluates surveyor performance through peer review, analysis of aggregate survey data, and feedback from organizations that have been surveyed. Such feedback is particularly important to the Joint Commission's internal quality assurance activities.

Survey Procedures

Although each survey varies according to the nature of an organization's programs and services, all surveys follow the same general process. The process leading to a formal survey begins when an organization applies to the Joint Commission for a survey. The length of the survey and the composition of the survey team are determined on the basis of information provided in an organization's Application for Survey. Survey fees are based on the number of surveyors on the team and the number of days they will need to complete the survey. Organizations can pay the full survey fee when billed or in two installments – half before and half after the survey. An organization is notified of its survey date approximately four to six weeks in advance of the on-site visit.

The next step in the process is the actual survey. On arrival, the surveyors usually hold an initial conference to discuss the survey schedule with representatives from the organization's administrative, major departmental, and medical or professional staffs.

Accreditation surveys are designed to enable the surveyors to assess the extent of an organization's compliance with Joint Commission standards. This is accomplished through one or more of the following means:

- A review of documentation of compliance provided by organization personnel;
- A review of information describing the manner in which a standard has been implemented or examples of its implementation; and
- Observations during the on-site visit.

During a survey, the surveyors also conduct interviews with anyone who wishes to communicate information about the organization to the Joint Commission. At such interviews, information may be presented by consumers and the public as well as by organization personnel and staff.

The surveyors always conduct a summation conference at the end of the on-site visit. At this conference, which should be attended by representatives of the organization's administration and staff, the surveyors report their preliminary findings. If deficiencies have been found, the surveyors may suggest measures that could be helpful to the organization in correcting the identified problems.

Tailored Surveys

An increasing number of health care organizations provide more than one category of services for which the Joint Commission has standards. For example, a hospital may have a long term care unit, or a long term care organization may provide organized medical and surgical services. In such instances, the Joint Commission tailors its survey process to meet the nature and needs of each organization. A tailored survey uses the standards specifically related to each of the services the organization provides. In the examples above, the organizations would be surveyed according to the applicable standards from both the *Accreditation Manual for Hospitals* and the *Long Term Care Standards Manual*.

Before a tailored survey is conducted, the organization receives a copy of each standards manual that will be used in the survey. The Joint Commission determines which manuals are applicable based on the information provided in the Application for Survey; on the application, each organization is to indicate all health care services provided under the aegis of its corporate governing body. A tailored survey is a single survey, conducted by a team of professionals chosen for their expertise in the services that will be surveyed. The organization receives a single accreditation decision based on the Joint Commission's evaluation of all health care services the organization provides.

Multihospital System Survey

The Joint Commission offers the *option* of a modified survey process for organizations that are part of a multihospital system. When a multihospital system elects the option of the modified survey process, the system's corporate office staff conducts a system orientation for the survey team to acquaint the surveyors with the system's organizational structure; at this time, the team reviews all relevant systemwide policies and procedures. To promote survey consistency, the same survey team is used, when possible, for all hospitals in a system. The hospitals in a system are surveyed in sequence when geographically feasible. After the surveys are completed, the team presents a summation of its corporate findings to the corporate staff. The modified survey process was designed to reflect the organizational structure of a multihospital system. However, each hospital within a system receives an individual survey and accreditation decision.

Systems that do not elect the option of the modified survey process are required to make available to the survey team any corporate bylaws, rules, policies, or procedures that affect the ability of individual hospitals in the system to comply with Joint Commission standards. This information can be provided at the corporate office or at the individual hospitals.

The modified survey process was adopted by the Joint Commission following an evaluation of its use in an extensive pilot program. The pilot program was part of a research project funded by the WK Kellogg Foundation of Battle Creek, Michigan. This project is described in the book *Organizations in Transition: A Report of the Joint Commission on Accreditation of Hospitals.*

Survey Findings

Regardless of the nature and type of survey, Joint Commission surveyors record the results of their findings on survey report forms once all pertinent information concerning an organization has been considered. For most accreditation programs, the standards manual serves as the survey report form. In the manuals, each chapter is in outline form, and the standards and required characteristics are followed by a five-point rating scale on which the surveyor indicates substantial compliance, significant compliance, partial compliance, minimal compliance, or noncompliance.

The surveyors use scoring guidelines to help them be as consistent as possible in assessing and ranking an organization's degree of compliance with the standards. The guidelines do not, however, preempt surveyor judgment. The Joint Commission is beginning to publish these guidelines to make explicit the bases for surveyor judgment that have been implicit for some time. The first of these publications is *Hospital Accreditation Program Scoring Guidelines: Medical Staff Standards.*

For new or revised standards that may require extended time for full and effective implementation, the Joint Commission uses a system called "implementation monitoring" to track an organization's progress toward compliance. Organizations that are found to be in less than substantial compliance with these standards will receive recommendations in the accreditation report. However, these recommendations do not constitute a contingency, nor do they affect an organization's accreditation status. Implementation monitoring enables the Joint Commission to provide to health care organizations additional assistance with standards interpretation and application. It also provides organizations with an indication of where further effort may be necessary before a standard can be fully and effectively implemented.

Once the survey report form has been completed, the surveyors provide a recommendation that an organization be accredited, be accredited with contingencies, or be denied accreditation. The appropriate documents are mailed to the Joint Commission, and the accreditation process begins.

Accreditation Procedures

The survey reports are analyzed by the Joint Commission's survey analysts. The analysts are responsible for validating the survey findings of each surveyor by comparing the scores on the survey report form with the accompanying documentation. The analysts record the collective, validated findings on an accreditation grid, on which the information that is necessary for making an accreditation decision is organized and summarized. The analysts discuss the results of their analysis with accreditation program staff, who confirm or revise the analysts' recommendation regarding accreditation, according to established decision rules and professional judgment. A final report with staff recommendations is then presented to the Accreditation Committee of the Board of Commissioners, which makes the accreditation decision.

An accreditation decision is made on the basis of the survey findings and any other relevant information. The major factors that affect accreditation decisions include evidence of overall compliance with standards, progressive advancement toward more complete compliance, and the absence of any serious impediment to assuring patient safety or maintaining acceptable quality of care.

Contingencies

If an organization is found to have areas of noncompliance with the standards that are serious but not severe or numerous enough to warrant nonaccreditation, the Joint Commission may accredit the organization with one or more contingencies. If an organization is granted accreditation with contingencies, the organization has full accreditation status, but it must achieve compliance with the standards in question before the next full survey is conducted; otherwise, except in unusual cases, it may lose its accreditation.

A contingency can be removed when the organization demonstrates substantial compliance with the standards in question. Such compliance is demonstrated when an organization submits an acceptable written report on its progress, or the Joint Commission conducts a survey visit that focuses on the areas of previous noncompliance in order to determine that the organization has achieved satisfactory compliance. The Joint Commission determines whether a progress report, a focused survey, or both will be necessary to address identified contingencies.

Nonaccreditation

If the Joint Commission determines that an organization should be denied accreditation, the organization is notified of this tentative determination. The organization is given 15 days in which to submit documentation in response to this notice. An organization may argue that the standards in question were not adequately assessed during the survey or may provide documentation that demonstrates compliance with the standards in question; or it may provide documentation which demonstrates that significant progress toward compliance has been made since the survey. After Joint Commission staff have reviewed the documentation, organization representatives may be invited to the Joint Commission to discuss the areas of noncompliance and any progress that has been made. Final staff recommendations are not presented to the Accreditation Committee until an organization has been given this opportunity.

Joint Commission staff review all material and information presented by the organization and recommend that the organization be accredited, with or without contingencies, or be denied accreditation. This recommendation, with supporting information, is then submitted to the Accreditation Committee. If, after reviewing all pertinent material and information, the committee decides to deny accreditation to the organization, the organization has a right to appeal the decision before it becomes final. The appeals procedures, which include access to a hearing and, ultimately, review by the Board of Commissioners, are explained in each of the standards manuals.

Confidentiality Policy

Regardless of an organization's accreditation status, the Joint Commission respects the confidential nature of survey findings. The strict Joint Commission confidentiality policy is included in the "General

Administrative Policies and Procedures" section of each standards manual. Except as required by law, specific survey findings are released only at the discretion of the surveyed organization. However, the Joint Commission does provide the following information on request:

- Whether an Application for Survey has been received from a particular organization;
- A list of organizations tentatively scheduled for survey, without indication of specific survey dates;
- Upcoming survey dates for a particular organization, after the organization has been notified;
- Whether or not a survey was conducted;
- Whether an organization is or is not accredited; and
- The accreditation history of a particular organization.

Duration of Accreditation

If an organization is found to be in substantial compliance with Joint Commission standards, it is awarded accreditation for three years (with or without contingencies). Approximately 18 months after its survey, an accredited organization receives a letter from the Joint Commission that emphasizes the importance of continuing self-assessment. The letter reminds the organization that correction of any recommendations it received in its last survey should be completed or well under way to avoid jeopardizing the accreditation award for the next full survey. At the request of an organization, the Joint Commission will conduct a full accreditation survey more frequently than once every three years.

Accreditation is not automatically renewed. An organization must undergo another full accreditation survey and demonstrate substantial compliance with the standards in order to renew its accreditation. Several months before the organization's accreditation is due to expire, the Joint Commission sends the organization an Application for Survey. After receiving the organization's application, the Joint Commission schedules a survey.

Summary

The Joint Commission designs its survey and accreditation processes to be as flexible and adaptable to changes in the health care field as possible. Because standards are the critical elements in assessing whether an organization should be accredited, it is essential that they be examined continually and revised as appropriate to reflect the state of the art in the practice and delivery of health care. ■

Chapter 3
The Standards

Because Joint Commission standards are used to assess whether an organization should be awarded accreditation, it is important to understand the philosophy underlying their development. Standards for maintaining quality exist in virtually all areas of business and industry and in all professions. Joint Commission standards are developed to maintain and improve the quality of care through providing a clear focus on the elements that are essential to the provision of high-quality care.

Standards Development

A standard is developed when there is an identifiable need to measure or enhance the quality of a particular aspect of health care or service. For example, new techniques, increased knowledge, or consumer demand for accountability can bring about the need to create new standards or to revise existing ones.

Such needs may be recognized by Joint Commission surveyors through their survey experiences, by Joint Commission staff members through their ongoing standards review, or by professional organizations or individual health care professionals in the field. The Department of Standards and the staffs of the accreditation programs work together to identify the need for, to describe, and to test substantive changes in standards and in the survey and accreditation processes.

When the need for change is valid, the standards development process is undertaken according to established procedures. If extensive changes are anticipated, a task force of experts in the area under consideration studies the issues and establishes principles to guide the development of new or revised standards. Generally, the findings of the task force are reviewed by the field. If the field review confirms that standards based on the guiding principles would improve the quality of care, the Department of Standards, in consultation with the task force, develops proposed standards.

In the course of developing standards, Joint Commission staff consider whether

- the proposed standards effectively address the identified need for new or revised standards;
- the proposed standards will improve the quality of care;
- implementation of the proposed standards will affect the cost of providing care;
- an anticipated increase in cost is worth any anticipated improvement in the quality of care;
- significant barriers to the implementation of the proposed standards exist; and
- Joint Commission resources and services (consultation, education programs, and publications) could help organizations to interpret and implement the proposed standards.

A draft of proposed standards may undergo extensive review both by Joint Commission staff and by thousands of individuals and organizations throughout the country. Those who participate in a field review include representatives of groups that the standards, if adopted, would affect. In addition, selected surveyors are asked whether the proposed standards can be surveyed. Joint Commission staff often modify proposed standards based on comments from the field and, in some cases, send subsequent drafts of the standards to the field for additional review.

The appropriate Professional and Technical Advisory Committee (PTAC) and the Standards-Survey Procedures (SSP) Committee oversee the entire standards development process. The committees review task force findings and recommended principles, where applicable, and approve principles for field review. The committees also review and, as necessary, modify proposed standards before and after they undergo comprehensive field review. When the SSP Committee deems the proposed standards acceptable, the standards are presented to the Board of Commissioners for approval. (See Table 1, Steps in the Standards Development Process, page 22.)

Standards development is a never-ending process. As organizations begin to address and comply with new or revised standards, Joint Commission staff review information about the standards, including aggregate and individual survey data. Particular attention is directed to progress in complying with standards designated for implementation monitoring. These reviews enable the Joint Com-

TABLE 1. Steps in the Standards Development Process

The standards development process is initiated when a need for new or revised standards has been identified. New and revised standards are usually adopted only after extensive review by the field. Minor or technical standards revisions may be adopted by the Board of Commissioners without field review.

1. The need for new or revised standards is identified.
2. If a major standards development effort is anticipated, a task force of experts is appointed, and Joint Commission staff conduct a literature review and provide background information to the task force. The task force usually proceeds with the development of appropriate principles. Alternatively, Joint Commission staff may conduct a literature review and draft standards.
3. The appropriate Professional and Technical Advisory Committee (PTAC) reviews the proposed principles or standards and makes recommendations to the Standards-Survey Procedures (SSP) Committee.
4. The SSP Committee reviews the proposed principles or standards and PTAC recommendations.
5. If approved by the SSP Committee, the proposed principles or standards are sent to the field for review.
6. In the case of field review of principles, Joint Commission staff, after considering the results of the field review, usually draft standards for task force review. The task force modifies the standards as necessary, and the standards are, with the approval of the SSP Committee, subjected to field review.
7. The results of the field review are reported to the PTAC, which reviews them and makes recommendations to the SSP Committee.
8. The SSP Committee considers the issues and modifies the standards as necessary. The preceding steps may be repeated until a reasonable consensus is achieved. The standards are then submitted to the Board of Commissioners for approval.
9. The Board of Commissioners usually either approves the standards or returns them to the SSP Committee for further development.
10. If approved by the Board of Commissioners, the standards are published in the appropriate standards manual, and the field is usually given six months* to achieve compliance with the new or revised standards.

**Through its implementation monitoring system, the Joint Commission extends this time period for certain specifically designated new or revised standards that may require additional time for full and effective implementation.*

mission to evaluate the effectiveness of new and revised standards as well as the need for any further refinement of the standards.

Standards Revision Project

In addition to its ongoing development and refinement of standards, the Joint Commission began a major project in 1981 to alter the basic nature and structure of the standards. Health care professionals require flexibility in devising new and effective ways of providing high-quality care in today's increasingly complex and sophisticated health care systems. Accordingly, the Joint Commission determined that its standards should be more general and less prescriptive in order to provide each organization with the opportunity to achieve compliance in ways that best suit its particular circumstances and methods of operation.

Specifically, the Joint Commission determined that its standards should

- relate as directly as possible to the quality of care and to the quality of the environment in which care is provided;
- reflect essential guidelines that every organization seeking accreditation should follow;
- represent a consensus on the state of the art;
- state, to the extent possible, objectives rather than mechanisms for meeting requirements; and
- be reasonable and surveyable.

Guided by these principles, the Joint Commission revises the focus and format of its standards to respond to the needs of diverse health care organizations and to the changes that are occurring in health care today.

The standards that were rewritten first were chosen because they are central to the administration and operation of hospitals and to the provision of high-quality care. These were standards for hospital governing bodies; management and administrative services; medical staffs; plant, technology, and safety management; quality assurance; and quality and appropriateness review in clinical support services. Although the Joint Commission began the standards revision project with standards for the Hospital Accreditation Program, it was clear from the outset that standards for all accreditation programs should emphasize competence-based practice and quality assurance. The revision of hospital standards served as a model for the revision of standards for the other accreditation programs.

The revised standards are intended to counteract any adverse effect on quality that may result from the overwhelming pressure on health care organizations to contain costs and to use resources appropriately and efficiently. To provide high-quality care, health care organizations must find ways to ensure that all individuals who provide patient care services are competent to do so and that the care provided throughout an organization constantly meets contemporary health care and environmental standards. Therefore, the Joint Commission is focusing on the effectiveness of the means by which organizations assess the competence of the individuals they allow to provide patient care services and on the effectiveness of an organization's quality assurance activities in identifying and resolving problems in patient care.

The Joint Commission's quality assurance standards and quality and appropriateness review standards provide a foundation on which competence and quality can be built. The quality assurance standards were rewritten to broaden the scope of the previous standards, which emphasized the performance of specific, discrete, and formal retrospective studies. The new standards emphasize the performance of ongoing, comprehensive, organizationwide quality assurance activities, focused on important aspects of care, to identify and resolve problems in patient care and performance and to capitalize on opportunities to improve care. As part of the organizationwide quality assurance program, all clinical support services are expected to monitor and evaluate the quality and appropriateness of the patient care they provide. The quality and appropriateness review standards were written to emphasize the performance of ongoing monitoring and evaluation activities and the importance of the actions taken, as well as the results of the actions taken, in response to these activities.

The revised plant, technology, and safety management standards illustrate the application of these concepts to other Joint Commission standards. The former standards for building and grounds safety and for functional safety and sanitation were rewritten and combined in the "Plant, Technology, and Safety Management" chapters of the standards manuals. The new standards reflect the state of the art in building and safety management as well as the many recent developments in health care engineering and technology. The standards emphasize the importance of competence and quality in providing a safe environment for patients and staff by identifying key aspects of life and functional safety that are to be carefully managed by qualified, capable individuals.

Directions for the Future

The Joint Commission historically has focused on the structure and process of health care delivery, but in the future, the accreditation process will also focus on the outcomes of care. The developmental process for this new direction will begin in 1987.

The Joint Commission has also begun developing standards to address the issue of undercare and to emphasize the importance of risk management activities to assure patient safety and quality assurance.

Summary

The Joint Commission Board of Commissioners, with input from PTACs, the SSP Committee, and the field, approves new and revised standards for all accreditation programs. Draft standards undergo extensive field review by thousands of health care professionals and representatives of consumer groups, associations, and government and private agencies.

Because of the many changes that have occurred in the health care environment, the Joint Commission is restructuring its standards to emphasize competence-based performance and quality assurance. ■

Chapter 4

Resources and Services

In its role as educator and consultant, the Joint Commission offers a variety of resources and services to health care professionals from a wide spectrum of organizations. Resources and services are provided to assist health care professionals in understanding the issues involved in providing high-quality care and in interpreting and implementing Joint Commission standards.

Resources

The Joint Commission's Division of Education comprises three departments that provide information and support services. The resources that are available are explained in the following sections.

Publications

The Department of Publications produces a variety of books and periodicals.

Standards Manuals. There are five standards manuals: the *Accreditation Manual for Hospitals*, the *Ambulatory Health Care Standards Manual*, the *Consolidated Standards Manual*, the *Hospice Standards Manual*, and the *Long Term Care Standards Manual*. The manuals are revised and updated as necessary, usually either annually or biannually.

Reference Materials. The Joint Commission publishes educational material on its standards and survey process and on quality assurance activities in specific settings and services. These publications are intended to assist health care professionals in understanding the standards and survey process and to provide practical examples of approaches health care organizations might take to achieve compliance with the standards. For example, the Joint Commission currently offers *A Guide to JCAH Nursing Services Standards*, *Quality Assurance in Long Term Care*, and a new series on the monitoring and evaluation of patient care. The first publication in the Monitoring and Evaluation Series is *Monitoring and*

Evaluation in Nursing Services; this publication is also included as part of the videocassette package *Consensus—JCAH Quality Assurance Standards: A Nursing Perspective*. To help health care professionals in state mental hospitals, freestanding psychiatric hospitals, and psychiatric units in acute care hospitals prepare for survey under the *Accreditation Manual for Hospitals* (*AMH*), the Joint Commission offers *Transition: Hospital Psychiatric Services and the AMH*. This audiocassette package includes the book *The Transition: Questions and Answers*, which can also be purchased separately.

The Joint Commission is, for the first time, publishing the scoring guidelines that are intended to improve surveyor consistency in scoring an organization's compliance with Joint Commission standards. The guidelines are being made available to the field because they express the intent of the standards and make explicit the bases for surveyor judgment that have been implicit for some time. The first of these publications, *Hospital Accreditation Program Scoring Guidelines: Medical Staff Standards*, was completed in late 1986; several others are scheduled for publication in 1987.

In addition, the Joint Commission publishes material in connection with its research projects. New and changing health care delivery systems are studied so that the characteristics of these systems can be examined and the need for the development of appropriate standards and survey processes can be investigated. The Joint Commission publishes the project findings and related material to communicate important information to the field. *The Hospice Project Report*, for example, describes the methodology and findings of the first large-scale study of the characteristics of hospices in the United States; the Hospice Project was funded by the WK Kellogg Foundation of Battle Creek, Michigan. Several publications have resulted from the Multihospital Systems Project, a cooperative effort of the Joint Commission and two multihospital systems that was funded by the WK Kellogg Foundation. These include *Multi-institutional Arrangements: A Review of the Literature*; *New Frontiers in Patient Care Assessment: Proceedings of the Multihospital Systems Invitational Conference*; and *Organizations in Transition: A Report of the Joint Commission on Accreditation of Hospitals*, which describes the methodology and findings of the project, and its companion publication, *Approaches to Patient Care Assessment in a Multihospital System: Report of the Sisters of Mercy Health Corporation*.

JCAH Perspectives. *JCAH Perspectives*, the official bimonthly newsletter of the Joint Commission, provides up-to-date information about the Joint Commission and its accreditation programs, including changes in standards, policies, and procedures; explanations of standards; and announcements concerning Joint Commission publications and education programs.

***Quality Review Bulletin* (*QRB*).** A monthly refereed journal, the *QRB* contains analytical and theoretical articles as well as practical descriptions of quality assurance activities and patient care evaluation techniques. In addition, special publications of the *QRB* offer collections of original and previously published articles on specific health care issues, such as *Maintaining Quality Under Pressure: The Dilemma of the Small Hospital, Risk Management and Quality Assurance*, and *Quality of Care for the Terminally Ill: An Examination of the Issues.*

PTSM Series. The Joint Commission publishes a Plant, Technology, and Safety Management (PTSM) Series, which consists of a handbook and periodic updates and monographs, to provide health care professionals with in-depth information on Joint Commission standards and issues related to plant, technology, and safety management. The series is applicable to all types of health care organizations. The *Plant, Technology, and Safety Management Handbook* provides information on Joint Commission standards in general and on PTSM standards in particular. The yearly updates might address, for example, information on developing an effective safety program; on managing hazardous materials and wastes; or on key items, probes, and scoring guidelines for PTSM standards. Each annual monograph contains a detailed analysis of a single PTSM issue.

For information on how to order publications, or to request a copy of the publications catalog, please contact the Joint Commission's Customer Service representatives.

Education Programs

The Joint Commission conducts numerous education programs throughout the United States for general acute-care hospitals, organizations that provide psychiatric services for adults or for children and adolescents, alcohol and substance abuse treatment and rehabilitation programs, ambulatory health care organizations, community mental health service programs, programs for mentally retarded/

developmentally disabled persons, long term care organizations, hospice programs, and home care services.

The Joint Commission offers national symposia, teleconferences, seminars, workshops, and custom-designed programs, which are designed by the Department of Education Programs to enhance health care professionals' understanding of accreditation and quality of care issues. Education programs are led by a variety of individuals, including Joint Commission staff and surveyors, outside consultants, active practitioners, and nationally recognized experts in various fields.

Certain programs, such as the "Program on Hospital Accreditation Standards," are specific to a particular accreditation program; they explain the intent of complex standards and provide examples of ways to meet the standards. Other education programs are designed to address specific health care issues that may be applicable to health care professionals in various types of organizations. For example, the "Plant, Technology, and Safety Management Seminar" provides safety professionals and others with a foundation for understanding the Joint Commission's PTSM standards for all settings. Another example is "Medical Staff Issues and the Changing Hospital Environment," which addresses concerns of and major issues that affect medical staffs. In addition, some education programs are designed for a particular group of health care practitioners. For example, "Assuring Quality Care in Nursing Services" provides nurse administrators who are already familiar with Joint Commission nursing services standards with the opportunity to integrate standards of practice into the monitoring and evaluation process.

The Joint Commission also custom designs programs to meet the educational needs of specific organizations. These programs, which are generally conducted on-site, provide a cost-effective, tailor-made approach to educating organization personnel.

All participants in the Joint Commission's education programs receive related resource materials. For more information on the programs, or to request a program calendar, please contact Customer Service at the Joint Commission.

Educational Resources

In 1986, the Joint Commission undertook improvement and enhancement of the educational resources that it offers to health care professionals. The Department of Educational Resources now offers on-site technical assistance for organizations interested in improving the effectiveness of their quality assurance and risk management activities. The on-site assistance is intended to assist organizations in resolving identified problems in their internal quality assurance systems and in improving the quality of care provided to their patients. Technical assistance services are provided by Joint Commission staff and outside consultants who have expertise in quality assurance and related issues. The cost of technical assistance services is calculated on a per-engagement basis according to the scope and nature of the engagement and the number and type of personnel involved.

The Department of Educational Resources has created a Resource Center to gather and catalog examples of successful approaches to meeting various accreditation standards. This collection consists of materials that demonstrate specific methods used by various health care organizations to meet the standards. By collecting, evaluating, and cataloging these materials, the Joint Commission is able to make them available for use by surveyors, in educational programs and publications, and by health care professionals from organizations seeking accreditation.

Additional information about technical assistance services and the Resource Center can be obtained by contacting the director of the Department of Educational Resources.

Services

The Joint Commission offers a number of special services for health care professionals from all types of organizations. The services offered include regional presurvey conferences for hospitals, on-site consultative visits, the Joint Commission Hotline, the Speakers' Bureau, and an audiovisual introduction to the Joint Commission.

Regional Presurvey Conferences

The Joint Commission's Hospital Accreditation Program offers regional presurvey conferences to hospitals through state and local hospital associations. A regional presurvey conference is held just before hospital accreditation surveys are conducted in a given geographic area and is intended to assist hospital personnel in preparing for survey. During the conference, a Joint Commission representative presents a summary of current activities, and surveyors explain the survey process. Much of the content of the conference, however, is determined by the hospitals themselves after they review the standards and decide what guidance they need. Usually, the Joint Commission asks hospitals to send in copies of written materials, such as specific policies and procedures, so that specific assistance can be given.

The cost of the conference is shared by the group of hospitals that have requested the conference. Requests for a regional survey conference should be made at least 60 days prior to the quarter in which the accreditation surveys are scheduled in the area. Additional information can be obtained from the Division of Accreditation Surveys.

Consultative Visits

The Joint Commission offers consultative visits to health care organizations that are interested in accreditation. The objective of these visits is to give organization personnel an indication of the organization's readiness for survey and to offer consultation regarding implementation of the Joint Commission standards. The typical consultative visit is conducted by one surveyor for one day, although additional time and extra surveyors are provided when necessary. During a visit, the surveyor discusses essential staffing and quality assurance functions and other areas as appropriate. The assessment of key accreditation issues includes document review and interviews with selected staff. In addition, the surveyor discusses the use of survey guidelines.

At the organization's discretion, the surveyor will conduct an orientation session to acquaint department heads with the Joint Commission and will present a summation briefing for organization management. After the consultative visit, the Joint Commission mails organization management a report of the surveyor's impressions and recommendations.

To request a consultative visit, organizations should contact the director of the appropriate Joint Commission accreditation program. The program director and organization representative can determine basic survey needs and decide on the date of the visit. The cost of a consultative visit is the same as the fee for a survey conducted by the accreditation program; that is, the cost reflects the number of surveyors and days required to conduct the consultative visit.

Joint Commission Hotline

The Joint Commission maintains a hotline service to help foster communication between the Joint Commission and its accredited organizations. The hotline is designed to answer those questions that are of an urgent nature and that require a timely response. The types of questions received through the hotline vary in nature and scope; callers often request information about standards, survey and accreditation procedures, and life safety requirements.

The toll-free hotline number is 800/621-8007; in Illinois, the number is 800/572-8089. A specially trained operator is on duty from 8:00 AM to 5:00 PM (central time) Monday through Friday. Calls received at other times are recorded and are answered during the regular working day.

The hotline has proved to be an important element in improving the Joint Commission's responsiveness to the field. To assure that the hotline remains open for the exchange of urgent information, the Joint Commission asks that callers use the general office number, 312/642-6061, for routine information.

Speakers' Bureau

Health care organizations are encouraged to take advantage of the Joint Commission's Speakers' Bureau to keep their members up-to-date about the accreditation process and Joint Commission standards. The speakers are Joint Commission surveyors and central office staff members. They will speak at conventions, meetings, conferences, and seminars sponsored by a variety of organizations.

Because the Speakers' Bureau tries to reach the largest possible audience at any given time, organizations within a given geographic area are encouraged to hold joint meetings when requesting a Joint Commission speaker. Requests for speakers should be sent in writing at least two to three months before the scheduled date of a meeting. Presentations generally last from 1 to 2½ hours and include a question-and-answer session. The request for Joint Commission speakers requires payment of all expenses and an honorarium.

Audiovisual Introduction to the Joint Commission

An audiovisual presentation is available at no charge to any organization seeking introductory material about the Joint Commission and voluntary accreditation. The color presentation is a 12-minute overview of the accreditation process, and it describes the benefits of voluntary accreditation and the resources that are available from the Joint Commission. The presentation is available in slide format and on VHS videocassette.

New board members or staff of health care organizations, staff of organizations preparing for an accreditation survey, and representatives of unaccredited organizations who are considering applying for a survey will benefit from this informative presentation. For more information on the audiovisual presentation, please write to the Corporate Relations Department.

Summary

The Joint Commission values its role as educator and consultant and encourages health care professionals to take advantage of the various resources and services available to them. Additional information on any of the Joint Commission's resources or services can be obtained by calling the general office number, 312/642-6061, or by writing to the appropriate department. ■

JCAH-4